The Ultimate Hair Weave Guide

Printed in the United States of America.

ISBN 978-0-9845268-0-2

How to order:

Additional copies of this book may be ordered directly from our website at www.Hair-Weave-Guide.com. Visit us online for updates and additional articles.

Please Note: The celebrity pictures throughout this book represent the variety of hair styles that can be created with the process outline in this book. They are not endorsements by the celebrity.

Contents

Introduction

This book is designed for anyone interested in looking great!

A hair weave is a relatively easy and non-invasive way to change your appearance. However, it is imperative that you take precautions to minimize the risk of damaging your natural hair and scalp if you are considering a weave for the first time. If you want to wear the latest hair styles and trends without the damaging effects of chemicals and excessive heat on your hair...this book is for you.

The Ultimate Hair Weave Guide was written by two experts with more than twenty years experience in perfecting hair enhancement techniques. Our first author is a former model, whose current corporate position demands a professional and flawless look every day. Over the years, she has perfected the process outlined in this book to apply and maintain her own hair weave.

The second author is her Hair Stylist of more than 15 years, who has dominated the stages of hair shows around the world with her cutting edge skills and techniques. She keeps her clients on track with the perfect cut, the right products and a maintenance schedule to fit their needs.

These experts will share with you a system that allows mega style and versatility while protecting and growing your natural hair.

Note: This book focuses on hair weave extensions because it is safe for home application and will cause the least amount of damage to your hair.

Hair Weave: What is it?

A Brief History...

Hair weave systems have been in existence since the early days of the Egyptians. According to the Encyclopedia of Hair, in the 1950's a hair dresser named Christine Jenkins developed a process of coarsely braiding the hair and sewing locks of hair directly onto a type of netting. This was an extremely expensive and time consuming process.

With all of Christine's efforts, the finished product was still quite bulky and looked unnatural – but it was the beginning of things to come.

Over time the quality of hair improved along with advancements in application techniques. In the 80's and 90's the demand for hair weaves made of soft, flowing human hair were all the rage. Stylists learned to create beautiful and completely undetectable hair styles, using small cornrows and applying the weft of hair directly onto the natural hair.

The first ten years of the 21st century brought about an enormous boom in the hair industry. Nearly 30% of all women use some type of hair weave, hair extension or add-on hair pieces to style their hair. Hair weaves have become a way to add versatility and style without damaging your natural hair with heat and chemicals.

Purchasing this book gives you a significant advantage over others. With practice and determination you will be able to style your hair like the celebrities – at a fraction of the cost.

In addition to saving tons of money at the salon, you can also EARN extra money by using these techniques on others (i.e., family and friends).

Note: The authors of this book do not encourage opening an unlicensed business of any type, however, most states do not require a license for braiding and extension/weaving services.

Is it possible to weave your own hair?

It is absolutely possible for you to weave your own hair, but first things first. There are two essential things needed when accomplishing any goal; and it is important that you acquire them prior to weaving your own hair. Interestingly enough, these two items cannot be purchased.

The first thing you must have before preparing to weave your hair at home is **vision**. You must visualize the finished product. Knowing the exact changes desired in your appearance is absolutely necessary. In order to make these decisions, it is helpful to have some type of visual aid. Whether it is a hair styling book, photos of your favorite celebrities, or computer generated images, you should spend the time to research and compare images.   It is important to make sure that the look is flattering for you. Be sure to consider hair length, texture and color. Envision yourself sporting a bold, new, trendy look and wearing it with pizzazz.

Celebrity hair style books may be purchased at bookstores, high-end supermarkets (in certain areas), or downloaded from the internet.

Another source of information is an honest conversation with your hair stylist. Who else is more qualified to offer an opinion about what looks best on you? Make an appointment for a consultation so that you have the uninterrupted attention of your stylist.

Be prepared with pictures and a list of questions you would like to have answered. Typically, hair stylists charge for consultations based on the amount of time spent with them. If you do your research, you will only need 20-30 minutes to get a professional opinion about what fits your facial shape, complexion and body type.

Now that you have a clear picture of which celebrity style you want and a professional opinion about what looks good on you, you're ready to proceed to the second acquisition.

The second thing you need before weaving your hair at home is **self-confidence**. You need confidence in your ability to get the job done. Have you ever shampooed and styled your own hair? Try to remember the hesitation you felt before getting started. You thought "What if my hair doesn't turn out right? Will I be able to go out in public?" You pushed past your doubts and tried it anyway. While it didn't look exactly like a professional did it, it was good enough to get compliments – right? The next time your stylist wasn't available and you styled your own hair it turned out a little better, because you <u>knew</u> you could do it.

Doing your own hair weave may be a little scary at first, but you have something you did not have the first time you styled your own hair. You have a step-by-step guide to read, re-visit, and understand before you start.

Our Hair Weave Guide walks you through the each step of the process. Our list of frequently asked questions provides additional support necessary to complete the job. It is said that "knowledge is power," however, knowledge has no power unless it is applied. It's going to take vision and self-confidence to actually apply these concepts.

You will also need self-confidence when sporting your new hair weave for the first time. Get ready for all types of comments. You don't owe anyone an explanation about your decision to improve your appearance. The haters are going to test you, so make sure you have a positive attitude about the "new look".

Hair does matter, so get ready for all the extra attention you will attract from the opposite sex. Your positive self-confidence and a new celebrity hair style will literally change your life.

Give yourself a pep talk, knowing that in the end you will look great for a fraction of the cost. In the following chapters we will walk you through the process of weaving your hair at home (with special attention to protecting your natural hair). With visualization, self-confidence, along with the Hair Weave Guide, you are now equipped – mentally and physically to proceed with your celebrity-style weave.

Failure is <u>not</u> an option.

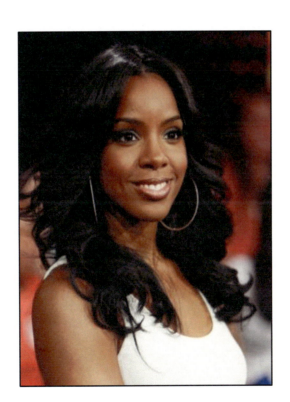

Who is the best candidate?

You are! Purchasing 'The Ultimate Hair Weave Guide' means you have a strong desire to look great while spending a minimal amount of money.

Hair extensions are worn for a number of reasons – the most common reason is to enhance appearance. In this age of plastic surgery, cosmetic dentistry and other appearance enhancements, women want to look their best from head to toe.

In addition to looking great, saving time is an added plus. A hair weave can be a great time-saver. Once curled, hair weaves can be maintained for up to a week before re-styling. It only takes minutes in the morning to freshen up your look. Wearing a hair weave can save a considerable amount of time getting dressed each day.

The typical candidate for a home hair weave is someone who has previously worn a weave. In this economy everyone is trying to cut back on expenses. The average hair weave can last anywhere from 4 to 8 weeks before it has to be removed and reapplied. During this time span maintenance must be done on a regular basis. This can be quite costly if you are having your weave serviced professionally. In the Hair Weave Guide we will teach you how to remove, tighten and service your own hair at home.

The term 'Professional Appearance' means looking your absolute best. Whether you work in the business sector or the entertainment industry, it is important that you look good. Celebrity-style hair weaves can be dressed up or toned down. Industries such as modeling, acting or anything in entertainment require exaggerated glamour. While the corporate environment or may require a toned down appearance. Either way you are an excellent candidate for a hair weave.

Have you ever wondered how you would look with a different hair color but were afraid to commit to a permanent change? Are you afraid of damaging you own hair by getting a high-lift color that requires bleaching? A good way to determine how a drastic change in hair color will look on you is to weave your own hair and try it. This way, if you don't like the result, you can always change the color without damaging your natural hair.

Do you have thinning hair? Maybe you have tried products that claim to grow or thicken the hair, but somehow nothing really works.

Maybe you've decided to wear a very short style because your natural hair has never grown past a certain length; or when it has grown, it's thin and stringy. Genetically, it may not be in the cards for you to have long or thick hair.

If you like the way you look in long lush wigs or hair pieces, this is your opportunity to have a long, natural looking care-free hair style without breaking the bank account. You are definitely a candidate for a hair weave.

Medications have many side effects. Persons taking certain medications may experience substantial hair loss. Ask your doctor or pharmacist if your prescribed medicine may cause hair loss. If the answer is "yes", you may walk away feeling helpless. You can take control of the situation. You have the option of doing a full head of hair weave or you may choose to enhance thinning areas by adding in a few tracks. Either way, you can take control of your appearance by weaving it yourself.

Homemakers want hair weaves to keep their youthful attractiveness and to maintain a sense of personal confidence. This type of woman takes care of the household and wants to feel beautiful by retaining or getting her youthful appearance back. She wants to feel that she is attractive to her husband, all of her friends, and most importantly to herself.

Working women desire to maintain their appearance so that they look and feel attractive within their peer group. A working woman is usually extremely busy and almost always pressed for time. She likely has children (possibly as a single mother) and only has time to interface with her peers on social occasions. A single working woman is very aware of her appearance as she may be pursuing a mate. Those are the times she wants to look and feel her very best.

Teenagers and young adults may have hair that just will not grow, yet they want to look like the divas they see in magazines and on TV. While teenagers may not be able to afford hair weaves regularly or over the long-term, they may try them for special occasions.

Bad haircut experiences can be devastating. Anyone who has had a bad haircut and would like to resume their original appearance is a good candidate for hair extensions. These people will wear them for a short period of time until their natural hair grows to the desired length.

If you can relate to any of these situations you are a good candidate for a hair weave.

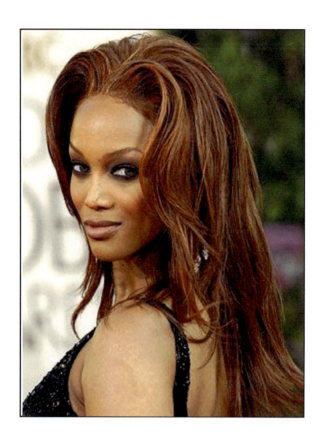

Who is not a good candidate?

Individuals with scalp irritations who experience chronic itching from dandruff, eczema or psoriasis may not be good candidates for hair weaves. In these instances the scalp must to be treated medically, therefore direct access is required. The hair weave could get in the way of treating the entire scalp area. Often times these conditions require frequent use of certain shampoos. The hair weave may loosen up considerably if shampooed more than once a week.

You are not a candidate for a hair weave if you are completely bald. You must have enough hair to attach the weft. Cancer patients who lose their hair because of chemotherapy treatment should seek other methods of hair replacement.

If you are more than 50 percent bald you would not be a candidate for hair weaving. There is not enough hair present to create the framework for complete coverage.

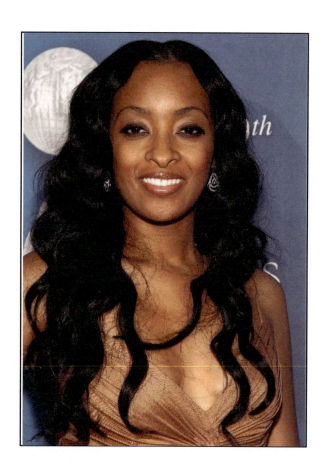

The Step-by-Step Process

The home hair weave process is simple and must be followed up with regular maintenance for the best results. While the entire process will be explained in detail in the following chapters – here it is at a glance:

1.   Select your style

2.   Purchase your hair

3.   Gather your supplies

4.   Prepare Your Hair

    a.   Remove any existing tracks
    b.   Shampoo / condition your hair

5. Braid your hair

    a.   Select a braiding pattern
    b.   Braid your hair
    c.   Secure the braid

6. Attach the hair to your head

    a.   Cut the weft
    b.   Sew the hair to your head

7. Get a great hair cut

8. Maintain your weave

    a.   Cleanse each week
    b.   Tighten tracks as needed

9. Remove and reapply as needed

Enjoy the compliments!

Supplies needed

The supplies needed for this process are very basic:

1. Hair: Machine or hand tied wefts (Note – hand tied wefts may eventually unravel)

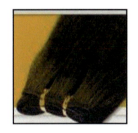

2. C-shaped Weave Needle

3. Nylon Weave Thread

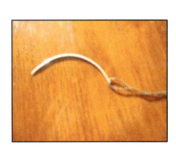

4. Hand Mirror

5. Small Scissors

6. Hair clip(s)

7. Comb / Brush

8. Seam Ripper (that's right)

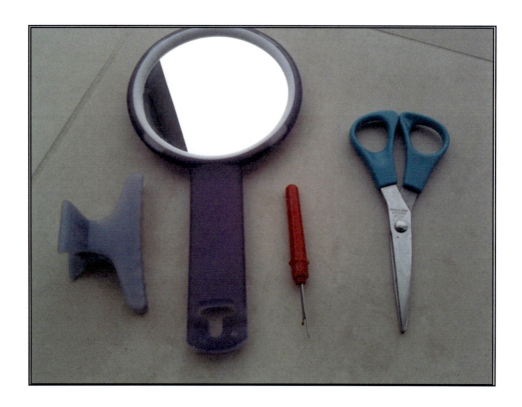

Tip: Be sure to purchase enough hair before you start the process. It is better to purchase a little more than you need to ensure you have enough to complete your style.

What type of hair should I use?

The type of hair you purchase will depend on the desired style.

Hair types range from poor quality synthetic hair to human hair of excellent quality.

What is Remy Hair?

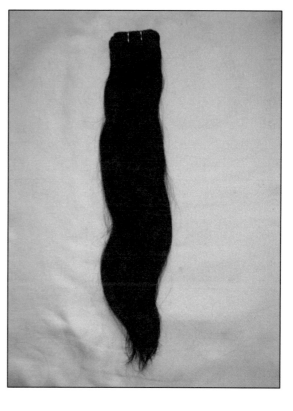

Remy (or Remi) Hair is one of the biggest buzz words in the hair industry today. You've probably seen all kinds of hair replacement companies big and small touting their Remy hair pieces. Some hair replacement vendors

may have even talked to you about the benefits of Remy hair, but have you ever wondered exactly what it really is?
Remy hair is human hair that is used in the production of hair pieces, wigs, hair extensions and a variety of hair goods products. The term Remy Hair is used on almost every hair product shipped from China – the biggest producer of hair goods in the world.

Simply speaking Remy Hair is human hair that is ventilated, tied or sewn with the cuticle of the hair all going in the same direction. The cuticle is the outer layer of the hair shaft and it is naturally a rough almost scaly surface. In production of human hair for hair goods the cuticle is usually smoothed, coated or compressed to make it smooth so the scales cannot catch on each other causing the hair to tangle and mat. While this process works well, the cuticle is still there and over time it is possible for the cuticle to swell and open up making the hair vulnerable to tangling.

To ensure the least amount of tangling the producers of hair goods make every effort to keep the hair cuticles going in the same direction to minimize the chances of tangling and matting. This enables the hair wearer to maintain the hair system with little problems and keep the hair looking natural with good movement.

The thing to remember is there isn't anything particularly special about Remy hair – it's just the industry standard. So be wary of vendors who concentrate on touting the great benefits of Remy hair or who try to sell you expensive Remy products. The fact is, Remy hair is not expensive to produce, and generally reputable suppliers will always offer this product.

If you are searching for a new hair supply retailer, don't worry so much about finding a company that advertises their hair as Remy. Concentrate on more important factors like overall quality and reputation of the vendor themselves. Do your homework and take the time to find a hair supplier that will truly work for you!

Human Hair

Most human hair used for weaving is shipped from Asia (China, India, and to a very small degree, Southeastern Russia). Lower-quality "human hair" extensions are often diluted with animal and synthetic hair to lower the price.

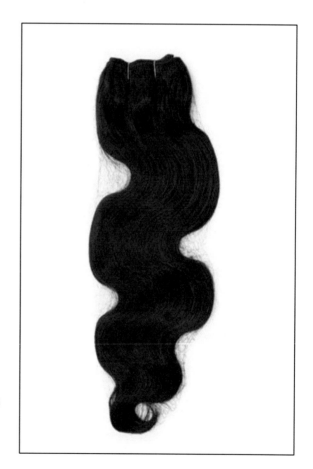

Human hair is, however, more versatile than synthetic hair because it can be colored, relaxed or curled with heating appliances just as one would do with his or her own hair. Since the weave wearer would want the hair to match the texture of her hair in its present condition (relaxed, curly, or straight), weave hair comes in a variety of textures: yaki (closely resembles relaxed hair texture), silky (resembling very straight Asian hair), European texture hair straight (Europeans generally do not sell their hair, therefore European hair usually comes from India or China), curly (ranges from tight corkscrew curls to the varying degrees of wavy), and crimped (very small, sharp waves).

There are different grades of hair. The highest grade comes from young donors, is gently processed, and of "Remy" designation. Remember, Remy means the hair's cuticles are facing the direction in which they grew.

The same maintenance that one would apply to his or her own hair should be applied to the human hair to keep it in good condition.

High quality 100% human hair is more expensive than hair mixed with other materials (synthetic hair is most common).

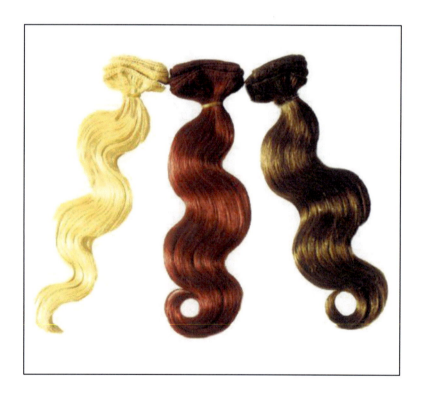

Synthetic Hair

Synthetic hair is made of a wide array of different synthetic fibers. Synthetic hair, just as human hair, comes in wefts. It does not last as long as human hair because it tends to easily tangle and frizz uncontrollably. There are, however, exceptions, and new technology facilitates the production of synthetic hair that minimizes these issues.

The quality of hair varies greatly, and if well maintained, synthetic hair can look as good as human hair. Synthetic hair is cheaper than human hair. The cost can range from $10.00 to $20.00 per package, depending on quality of hair, length, brand etc.

Heating appliances such as curling irons and blow dryers should <u>not</u> be used on synthetic hair.

There are newer types of synthetic hair from certain brands that claim to allow styling with lower temperatures of heating appliances.

Generally, people should steer clear of such claims because the golden rule with synthetic hair is that heat is not an option.

For this reason synthetic hair is <u>not</u> recommended for hair weaving.

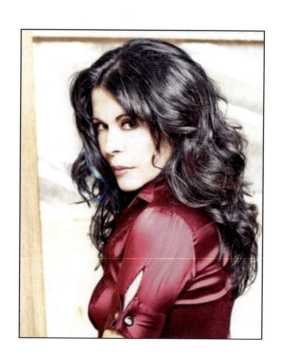

How much to purchase

The amount of hair needed will depend on the style you want. For example: If I have hair to my chin line and I want hair to extend to my bra line (about 18" long), I might need 5 or 6 tracks/wefts depending on my current haircut. If I have hair to my shoulders that is thin and stringy and I want it thicker and more luscious but keeping same length, I might need 2 or 3 (or more) tracks/wefts.

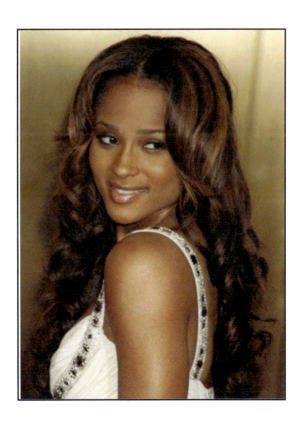

Preparing your natural hair

I. **Remove any existing hair tracks (if necessary)**

Step 1 – Pull any existing hair weave up into a ponytail at the top of your hair. If you have a short style put clips around your head. Take the last track in the back and release it from the pony tail. Using your fingers, feel the different between the thread and your own hair. If necessary, use a hand a mirror while standing with your back facing your bathroom mirror you so you can actually see the track.

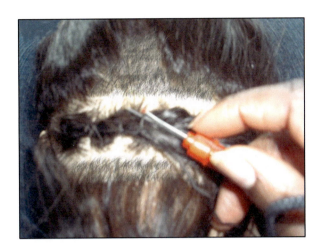

Slip the seam ripper under the thread loop holding the weft to the braid and push through one piece of the thread at a time (careful not to cut your natural hair).

Step 2 – Picking up where you cut the thread, pull (or lift) the remaining thread with your fingers. Continue to the end of the row. You may have to make extra cuts if you find knots, usually at the end. Once cut you can easily remove the weave.

Step 3 – Use your fingers to remove any remaining thread tangled in the braid.

Step 4 – Loosen the braid. Start at the end of the braid and use the comb's teeth or tail to separate the braid. Pull down until it starts to unravel.

Step 5 – After you have removed the entire braid you might see a clump of hair or build up at the root. Use your comb to gently comb through the clump starting at the ends and working down.

If the clump of hair is tough to move, use your fingers to rub it back and forth loosening up the ball of hair before you comb through it.

Step 6 – Continue removing each braid in this manner until they are all out.

Step 7 – Comb through your entire head of hair before you move on to washing and conditioning.

> **Tip:** Do not leave braids in more than 8 weeks. After that length of time the chances of tangling and breakage are much higher.

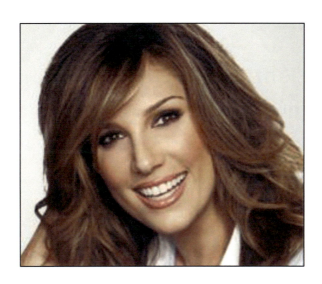

II. Shampoo your hair

Your hair is very delicate, so use the gentlest shampoo available that meets your hair's needs.

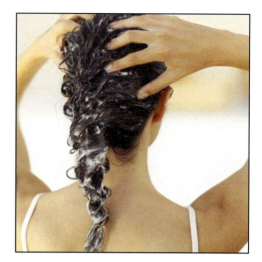

Note for Black Hair: Use shampoo sparingly because squeaky clean isn't always a good thing.

Step 1 – Gently detangle your hair with a wide tooth comb. (Skipping this step may cause your hair to lock-up later in the process.)

Step 2 – Saturate your hair with warm water before you apply the shampoo.

Step 3 – Use a dime or quarter-sized amount of shampoo depending on the length of your hair. Work it into a lather. Concentrate on your scrubbing your scalp.

Remember, shampoo is for the scalp and conditioner is for the hair.

Step 4 – Massage your scalp deeply to invigorate it and loosen flakes that might be there.

Step 5 – Thoroughly rinse your hair until all traces of shampoo are gone. This should take about 1 ½ to 2 minutes. Part your hair and check to make sure all the shampoo is out.

Step 6 – Gently squeeze the water out of your hair.

Tip: Do not use hot water to wash your hair. Warm water is best for shampooing and rinsing.

III. Condition your hair

An important part of caring for your hair is using a quality conditioner. Shampoo gets your hair clean but conditioner makes it look healthy.

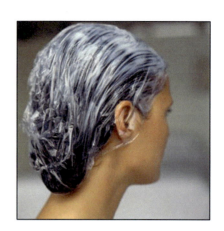

Step 1 – Apply a generous amount of conditioner from roots to ends. Concentrate on the last 1/4 of the length since this is the oldest part of your hair. Try to avoid getting conditioner on your scalp, especially if you have flake issues.

Step 2 – Leave conditioner on according to instructions. For optimal conditioning use a plastic cap and heat for a deep penetrating treatment.

Step 3 – Rinse, but don't over rinse. You want to leave a tiny bit of conditioner in your hair.

Step 4 – Gently squeeze and blot the water from your hair.

Step 5 – If time and your hair texture allow, the best option is air drying. If not use your blow dryer on a cool setting.

Never skip conditioner after shampooing your hair. Moisture must be put back after the oils have been stripped out with shampoo.

Tip: To make your comb glide through your hair mix a good hair serum with your leave-in conditioner. Apply it before you comb for unbelievable results!

IV. **Leaving your hair slightly damp makes it easier to braid.**

If you are planning to wear a part or bangs, now is the time to part off those sections so that as you are braiding the hair you can work around those areas.

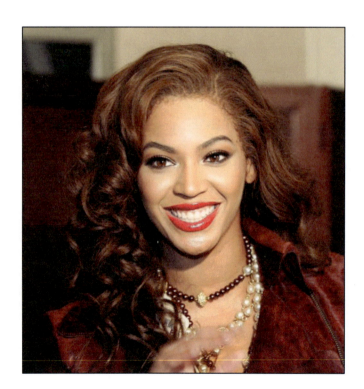

How to braid your own hair

Learning how to braid your own hair takes a little patience and coordination. Just remember practice makes perfect.

The first step in braiding hair is to comb it smooth. Make sure you remove every single knot and tangle – or it will come back to haunt you later on in the process.

Some people like to braid their hair while it is wet, but if you have particularly thick or long hair, your braids may take a long time to dry. I prefer to start with dry hair, and spray on a leave-in conditioner to mildly dampen each section just before braiding.

For very <u>STRAIGHT HAIR</u> you may need to use a hair wax that is based on distilled water (not oil) to prevent slippage.

For very <u>CURLY HAIR</u> you should use a moisturizer that does not break down too soon such as a hair food.

Remember precise braiding makes the style last – not pulling hard from the scalp. Pulling too hard from the scalp only leads to pain and hair loss.

After you've planned your braiding pattern, part a section of your hair that you want to braid. Clip your other hair up and out of the way so that you have a clear path to follow.

Tip: You can learn to braid by using three pieces of string or rope laying flat on a table. Once you understand the concept, it's easy to make the transfer to braiding hair. Once you are adept at making the braid you will want to hold all three sections in your hands to increase your braiding speed.

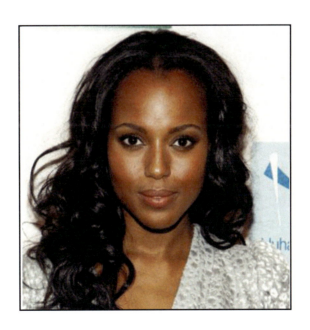

Take a small section of hair
where you want the cornrow
braid to begin and comb the
section smooth.

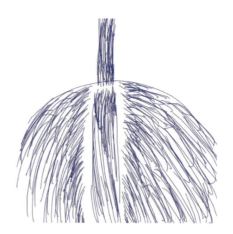

Make 3 strands out of the hair
you've separated in order to
begin the row. Careful not to
pull too tight near the
hairline.

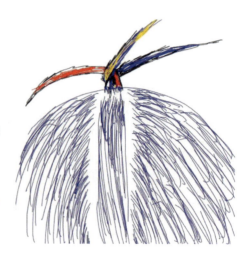

Cross the right hand section
under the middle section. The
original right hand section is
now the middle section.
Using your forefinger add new
hair to the middle section.

Pull all the sections away from
each other to keep the hair
snuggly taut throughout the
braiding process.

Cross the left hand section under the middle section. The original left hand section is now the middle section. Using your forefinger to add new hair to the middle section.

Make one or two "stitches" of a regular braid. Continue to pick up some hair from the rest of the section you've parted.

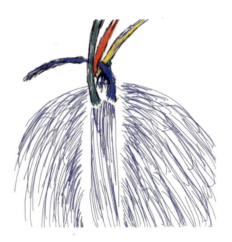

Continue the process alternating right and left sections under the middle section, tightening each stitch as you make it.

Braid all the way to the very end of the hair.

Braiding won't be easy the first time you try it but with just a little bit of practice you will quickly become a braiding expert.

Securing the braid

Securing (or tacking down) the braid creates a stable foundation for the weft of hair. You are simply tacking down the braid and sewing the excess braid (that extends past the head) underneath the cornrow.

Take the end of the braid and lay it down along side itself so the section that is not attached to the head can be sewn adjacent to the cornrow. Use the curved needle and thread to sew the braid onto itself using a looping stitch.

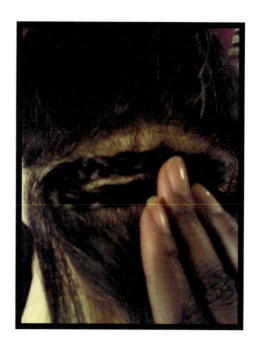

This is done by slipping the curved needle under each row of braid and pull through to the other side.

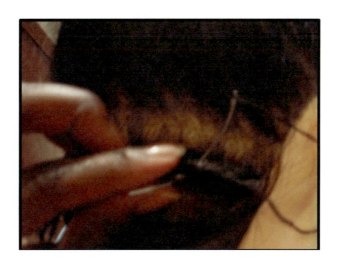

If your hair is short or slippery you can add extra security by looping the loose thread around the needle before pulling it completely through to make an anchor.

Repeat this process until you reach the entire length of cornrow and the loose end of the braid has been sewn onto itself.

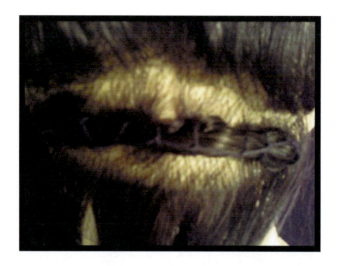

Cut the end of the thread about three inches away from the scalp. Tie down the two loose strings in a double knot and cut off any slack.

Secure each braid in this manner before attaching the hair as you complete your weave.

Now you're ready to attach the weft of hair onto the braid.

Use the same loop (and anchor) stitch to attach the hair to the braid.

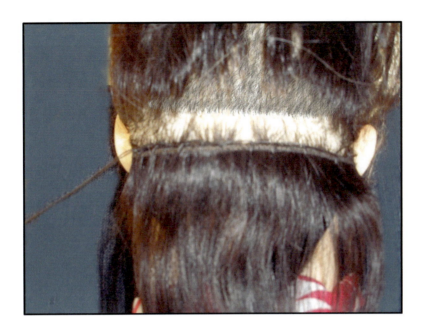

Go over the same spot a few times with the needle and thread when you start the track to secure it properly. Do the same thing when you get to the other end of the cornrow.

Braiding patterns for weaving

There are many braiding patterns to choose from; however, when you are maintaining the weave yourself, you want a pattern that is easy to keep tight and flawless.

Circular / Snake Patterns – are almost impossible to braid yourself (you would need rubber arms). Also, as your natural hair grows, it is not possible to tighten just one section/area.

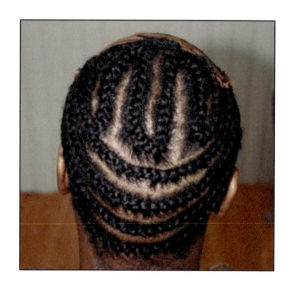

All the hair must be removed and the hair completely re-braided to tighten the style.

Vertical Braid Patterns – Vertical braids down the back of the head are usually joined together down the middle of the head or across the bottom at the base of the neck. Either way seems to create an unnatural (bulky) hump. This is less noticeable if you are attaching curly hair as opposed to straight hair.

Recommended Patterns For Home Weaves

There are three main patterns to use depending on the style and whether there will be a part (middle or side) or bangs swept to the side.

Part in the center:

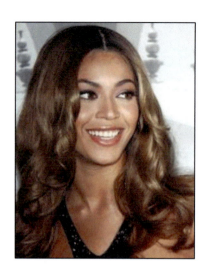

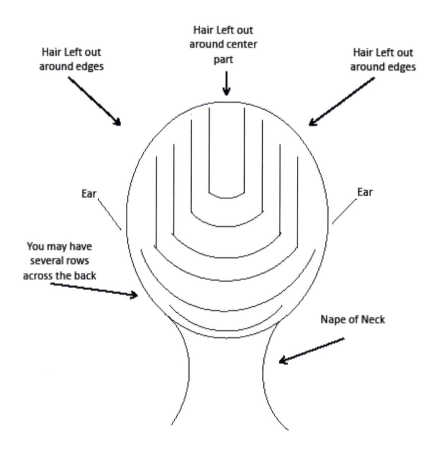

Hair Left out around center part

Hair Left out around edges

Hair Left out around edges

Ear

Ear

You may have several rows across the back

Nape of Neck

Part on the side:

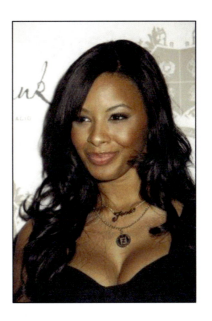

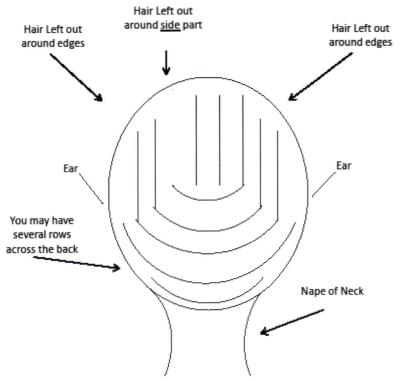

Hair Left out around <u>side</u> part

Hair Left out around edges

Hair Left out around edges

Ear

Ear

You may have several rows across the back

Nape of Neck

Front Bangs:

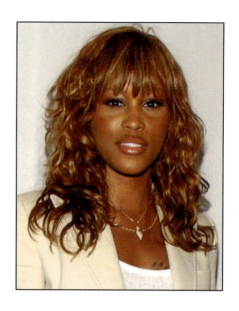

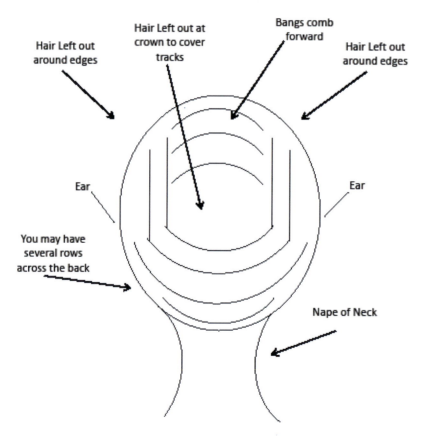

Hair Left out at crown to cover tracks

Bangs comb forward

Hair Left out around edges

Hair Left out around edges

Ear

Ear

You may have several rows across the back

Nape of Neck

As each track is braided and secured, the wefts are sewn to them and then your own crown area hair is blended with and combed over to cover the extensions.

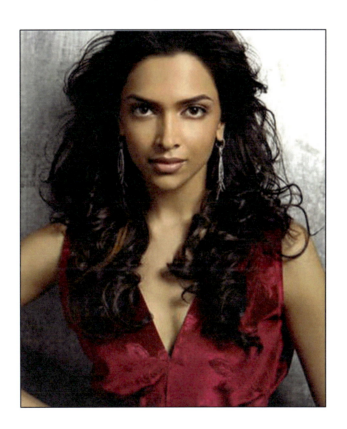

Attaching the hair to your head

With your natural hair clean and dry, your braiding pattern selected, you are ready to braid and attach the wefts of hair. You will repeat three basic steps for each track: 1) braid your hair; 2) secure the braid with thread; and 3) attach the hair.

You will cut and attach the hair weft as you complete each braid.

When attaching the hair, its best to start at the back of the head and work your way up to the front.

Start with the back at the nape of the neck. Make a part across (left to right) about an inch or two from the hairline at the base of your neck.

It is very important that the part is STRAIGHT.

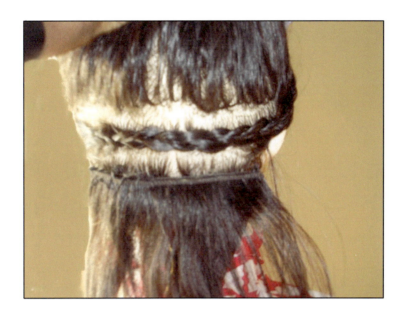

The hair will not hang naturally if one side is higher than the other. One way to ensure the part is straight is to stand in the bathroom with your back toward the mirror on the wall, use your hand mirror to check the part. Re-part and re-check until you get it completely straight – it just takes practice.

I find it easier to braid from the left side to the right side (I'm right-handed). Continue braiding until you run out of hair to braid (don't stop at the hairline).

Next secure the braid with thread using the instructions in previous chapter.

Now you are ready to attach the hair to the secured braid. First, take the hair weft and hold it against the braid to measure the length needed, holding your finger in the place where it should be cut.

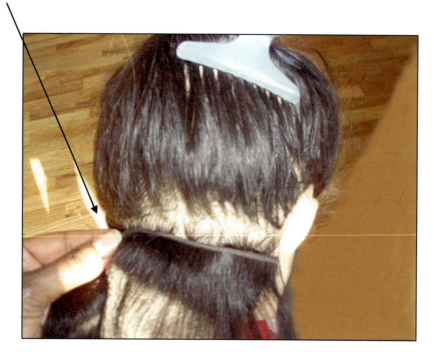

It is best to cut the hair after the braid is complete so that you can measure the exact length (you don't want to waste the hair).

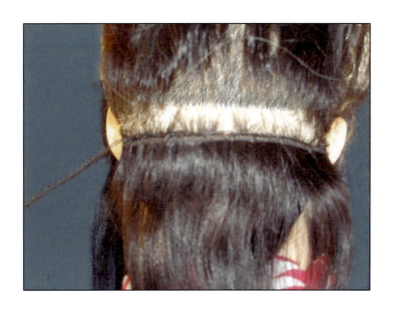

Start attaching the hair using the looping stitch (I usually anchor the hair to the right side sewing toward the left). Each stitch should be no more than ½ inch apart. If you have larger gaps between stitches, the weft will buckle between the stitches when you wash your hair.

Tight, close stitching keeps the hair flat and flawless.

Make the next part about 1½" higher than the last and repeat the steps above:
Braid – Secure – Attach.

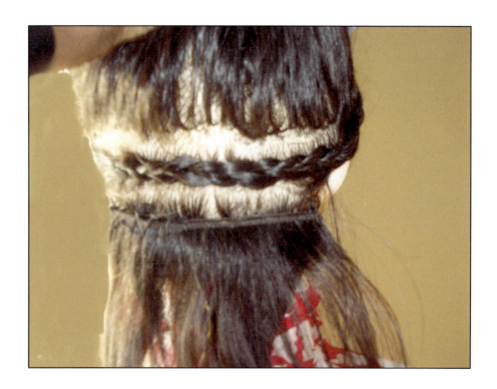

Tip: If you are only adding 2 or 3 tracks for volume or length, leave room for your natural hair to blend between the tracks.

SUMMARY / TIPS:

- Check each part using your hand mirror to be sure the part is straight – BEFORE braiding the hair.

- Secure each braid with thread.

- As you are sewing the hair weft to the track, keep the stitches very close together ½" or less, especially at the top of the head and around your part.

- If you have a part or bangs, be sure to leave enough of your natural hair out at the crown to cover the tract around your part.

- Keep your braids 1½" to 2" apart. If you have larger gaps between the braids three to four inches, your natural hair will begin to poke out over the weeks as you wash your hair.

(This is fine if you are only adding a few pieces for volume.)

If you perfect these tips your hair will last and be flawless!

A full head of hair for me is about 8 rows of hair in the horseshoe shape including the U braid around my part. Now that I have perfected this process I can complete a full head in about four hours.

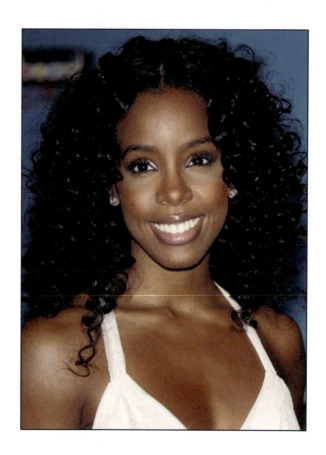

Getting the right cut

The success and failure of a great looking weave hair style depends heavily on the haircut. Just as a great haircut on your natural hair is the foundation for the style, so it is with your hair weave.

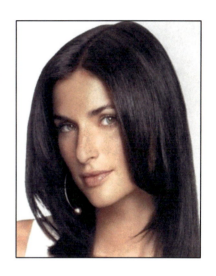

We recommend you go to the professionals for this part of the process.

After you have successfully completed the tracks, we strongly suggest that you see an experienced hair stylist. Someone who does great cuts with natural hair is usually someone who understands the importance of texture, style and weight distribution.

Unfortunately, the ideal person to cut your hair weave may not be your regular stylist. Your regular stylist may or may not have experience cutting hair extensions.

In order to make sure you hire the right stylist you may need to do a bit of leg work.

First, if you have never seen your stylist cut weaved hair, that's a pretty good indication that she does not have the required experience. Start by noticing other stylists in the salon. If you see a stylist doing hair weaves (that look great) regularly when you're at the salon, ask your stylist if he/she minds if you have a consultation with them.

If not, ask someone who wears an attractive weave style, who does their hair. Whether it is a referral or another stylist in your regular salon there are some key questions you should ask before making the appointment.

The four key questions you should ask are:

1. **How long have you been cutting hair weaves?**

   This helps you to determine whether or not this stylist is a great haircutter, who can cut different styles on a weave, or if they are limited to one or two looks. Make sure they are able to be versatile with hairstyles.

2. **What tools do you use when cutting a hair weave?**

    A good haircutter should use scissors and either a razor or thinning shears, possibly all three.

3. **What sets you apart from other hair cutters?**

    This is where they may share their credentials, cutting and finishing classes or higher levels of training for their craft. If this question irritates the stylist, you may want to thank them for their time and move on to your next option. Any hair stylist who is highly trained does not hesitate to brag about their accomplishments.

4. How much is this going to cost me?

The price should be comparable to the price of a regular haircut in your area. Remember that you get what you pay for. If the price seems too low, be suspicious. If it's a few dollars more, it could be that you have a very experienced hair stylist who is confident in their work.

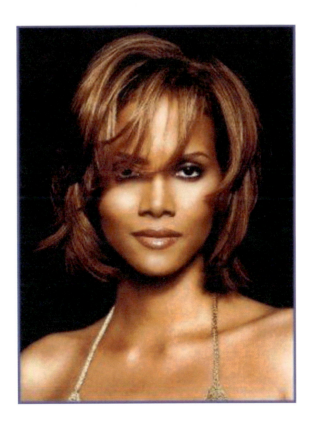

How much is this cut worth?

How to style your celebrity hair

When choosing a celebrity-style hairdo, there are some basic things you need to consider. Your hair style should compliment your body. <u>Balance</u> is the word. A big coiffure emphasizes a small lady's statue by making her head seem enormous and her body even smaller.

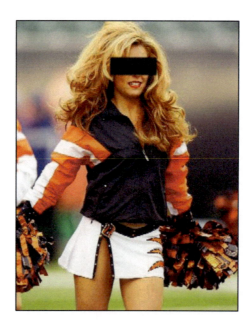

Similarly, a small coiffure on a big individual draws attention to her body by shrinking the appearance of her head. As we age, gravity takes hold softening our features and silhouettes. A severe hairstyle often emphasizes this and makes you look older. I don't believe that length or the lack of length influences a styles' severity as much as volume. Yes, Poker straight waist-length hair with a center part is harsh, while long wavy hair with plenty of body is gentler. The adage to keep in mind is that as you age, go softer.

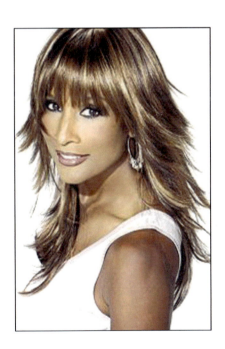

When choosing the right style, remember to ask the advice of your professional hair stylist when you go in for the cut and consultation. They can advise you on styles that will compliment your facial shape. Once you have decided on a hair style be sure to observe the tools used by your stylist as well as the direction of the curl patterns used to achieve the hairstyle.

Hairstyling tools

There are many hairstyling tools that work like magic to give your hair that flawless look you desire. Hairstyling tools are essential to have, especially if you want to look your best. There are a variety of hairstyling tools on the market that range from inexpensive to very expensive. Stay with the mid-range pricing for non-professional use.

In order to re-style your celebrity hairdo at home you will need the following tools.

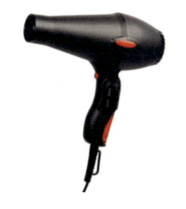

Blow dryer – is essential to dry and loosen the hair, also to eliminate frizz (the higher the speed, the smoother the hair) and create body and volume.

Hood dryer – is used to dry the tracks and prepare hair for blow drying.

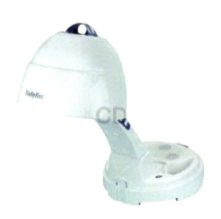

If chose not to sit under a hood dryer you may shampoo the night before and allow tracks to dry naturally, but the hair should be kept straight while drying over night. Try pulling it into a ponytail.

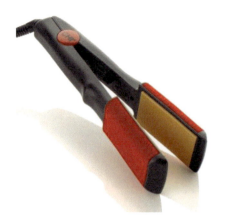

Flat Iron – is used to straighten hair for long sleek looks with minimum curl and body.

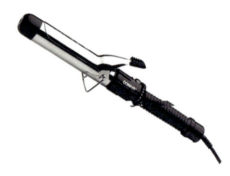

Curling Irons – are used for styles requiring more body and/or curl.

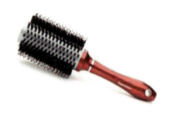

Round brush – is used after hair has been dried. With use of the blow dryer, the round brush adds lift to the hair.

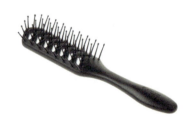

Flat (vent) Brush – may be used to dry and smooth the hair with use of the blow dryer.

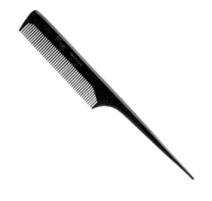

Rat tail comb– is used for sectioning the hair to be curled or flat ironed.

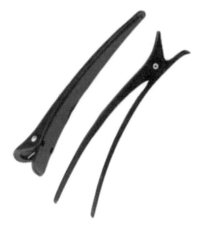

Hair clips – are used to clip away the sections that are not being curled.

Step-by-Step Styling
for Celebrity Hairdos

Step 1 Shampoo, condition and rinse hair thoroughly.

Step 2 Apply mouse, styling lotion, or gels to natural hair only (if applicable) leaving your hair extensions free of product.

Step 3 Mold hair and sit under hood hair dryer until tracks are completely dry.

Step 4 Blow dry hair to loosen from roots to ends adding movement and texture (Use vent brush for flat styles or round brush to lift hair for more volume).

Step 5 Flat Iron or curl hair according to style desired.

Step 6 Brush hair to create a finished look (in some instances you may use fingers to lift hair in key areas).

Step 7 Lightly spray hair with medium hold (pump) hairspray for lasting results.

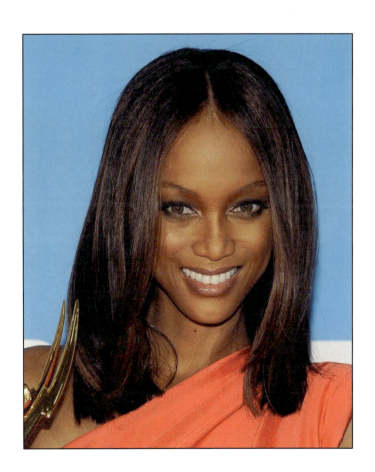

How to keep your style fresh?

My stylist is always amazed at how fresh and new my weave looks after 6, 8 or even 12 weeks. Each week I cleanse (shampoo and condition) my hair thoroughly and my stylist flat irons it straight for me.

MY SECRET: Before shampooing, I remove and replace one track each week (weft and braid). This only takes about 20 minutes or so. The last row in the back (at the nape of the neck) will loosen first because of the tension from brushing and styling – so start with the back row. At times there may be a track in the front that needs to be replaced sooner and I will divert from the normal order.

Begin this process of removing and replacing the tracks after wearing the weave for three to four weeks.

If you wear a full head (8 or 9 rows) as I do, you will want to do this each week. If you only have 3 or 4 rows across the back to add length or fullness to your hair, it may not be necessary each week. Check for looseness and do what works best for your style.

The goal is to prevent the obvious gap between the track and your scalp, as a result of your new growth. This is most noticeable in the very front and the very back of the head and it gives your style a wig-ish look.

Braiding you hair in the patterns suggested in this book will make it easy to keep your style looking new and fresh. If your hair is braided in continuous or snake cornrows as opposed to the individual rows, the entire weave must be removed in order to tighten.

Brush your hair before you go to bed and sleep in a silk cap. While brushing, be sure to hold the tracks (with one hand) as close to the head as possible, use the other hand to brush through the hair. This prevents pulling and jerking on the natural hair.

Use heated styling tools carefully. If your extensions are made from a low quality synthetic, then it is unwise to blow dry or use heated styling tools. If you have human hair, you should be able to treat them in much the same way as your natural hair.

Shampoo once a week. Shampooing your weave too much can dull its shine, but not shampooing it enough can cause it to clump at the ends and lose its swing and bounce. Once-a-week washing strikes a perfect balance. When shampooing, always comb your weave free of tangles while the hair is slathered with conditioner, so the comb doesn't pull and snag at the hair.

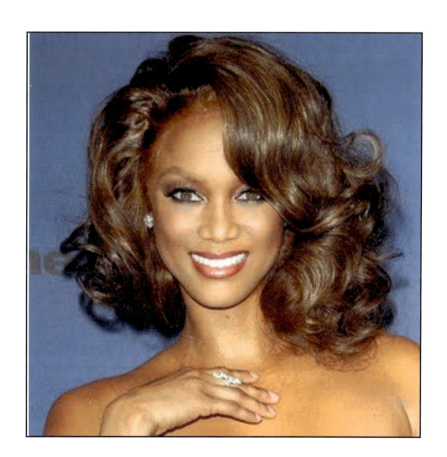

Tips for Maintaining your hair weave

Your hair weave requires thorough maintenance; otherwise you may ruin it before its time. You must be careful with everything from combing to washing. Common tips you should keep in mind while dealing with weaved hair are as follows:

1. Normally you comb your hair from head to the ends, but to comb weaved hair you should start from the end and then gradually move upwards to the head. All while holding the track in place.

2. Brush before you wash or shampoo your hair and rinse between the tracks to remove the residues.

3. You should shampoo the hair every week, but no more than two weeks between shampoos. Always use mild water while washing the hair, as too hot or too cold water may lock the hair at the base.

4. Avoid using harsh products for washing, styling or conditioning.

5. Alcohol based product will tarnish the sheen of the hair and you should not use them.

6. Do not skip regular tightening touch-ups (this varies depending on care of weave and/or growth rate of hair) typically every other shampoo.

High tension areas may need to be tightened every week.

7. Use of cotton pillowcases and sheets may adversely affect the shine of your hair; use a silk or satin scarf to wrap up your hair.

8. During blow-drying, you have to apply higher temperature to straighten and dry the hair. Use variable temperatures for the natural and commercial hair.

9. If you wish to swim, either use a swim cap or saturate and rinse the hair by applying a cream rinse before plunging in and a detoxifying shampoo and moisturizing conditioner afterwards.

10. While you may doubt the details involved in removing the weave, it is better to have a friend cut the tracks

out for you especially in the back of your head until you are comfortable with doing it yourself.

Dirt, sweat, styling products and natural oils are some of the ingredients that interfere with clean hair condition.

You should regularly shampoo and condition the hair to keep it clean. Excessive use of styling products have been shown to shorten the longevity of hair extensions.

Thus, proper care is needed to keep the different types of hair problems associated with hair extensions at bay.

Tips for Maintaining your natural hair

To maintain your natural hair while wearing the weave, it is important that you pay attention to what is happening with your natural hair when you remove the tracks for a tighten up. Here's a checklist of things you should watch for:

1. Is your natural hair properly cleansed and conditioned?

    After the 6 to 8 week period of wearing weave, do you notice a build-up of dirt and debris?

If so, you may not be shampooing and rinsing the hair thoroughly.

2. Make sure you are not over-processing your natural hair chemically while wearing the weave.

    <u>Hint</u>: Only relax or retexture the hair that is left out around the hair line.

3. If wearing a part, alternate the sides periodically.

4. Until you get the feel of cutting your own tracks out, have someone cut them for you so that you do not snip into your braided hair.

5. Use leave-in conditioners.

6. Give yourself a hot-oil and strengthening treatment in between weaves.

7.   Never perm or color hair in between the tracks.

8.   Touch-up (perm or color) hair lines no more than once every 4-6 weeks.

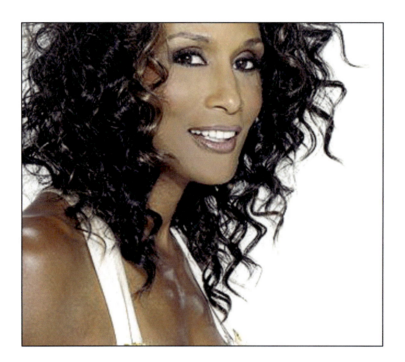

Top Secret celebrity tricks

1. Shampoo, condition and dry the (purchased) hair before attaching to your head.

2. If you are wearing a full head weave, leave the least amount of natural hair out around parts or edges to cover the tracks. Use a flat iron to blend the natural hair with the weave hair.

3. If you are planning on styling your hair in an up-do. Do not braid all the way to the edge of your hair line (on the sides). See below:

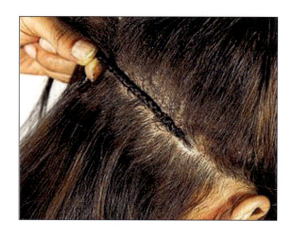

4. If you are only adding hair for length or volume do not start at the nape of the neck. Start closer to the ears.

5. Tack down your braids before applying the wefts of hair. This will create a flat weave that will last longer.

6. To keep your style looking fresh and tight, after three to four weeks remove and reapply one row per week (hair weft and cornrow).   Start with the last row at the nape of the neck and work your way to the top, it takes about 20–30 minutes to remove and reapply. This prevents the wig–ish look caused by your natural hair growing out.

7. Learn to comb and brush your hair while holding the hair weft close to your head with one hand. This will prevent premature loosening.

8. Wrap your hair in a silk scarf before going to bed at night. This will keep the tracks lying flat and in position. The silk scarf also won't snag the hair or break the ends.

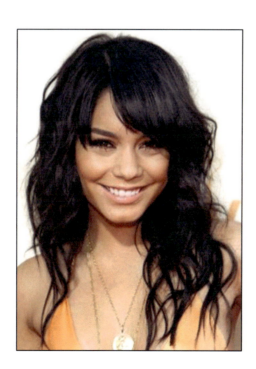

Recommended products

There are many brands to choose from and various manufacturers who meet the demand of great hair care for natural hair and hair extensions. Their products have been long standing and maintain integrity.

The products recommended will depend on the texture of the hair you are wearing.

For curlier hair types, you should use shampoos and conditioners formulated for curly hair. They tend to provide more moisture and detangling agents.

For the straighter hair it is important that the products are recommended for relaxed hair. These products contain ingredients to close the hair cuticle down allowing it to lay smooth, shiny, and in the same direction.

Many professional lines have long term reputations for great performance on ethnic hair.

To name a few:

Aveda

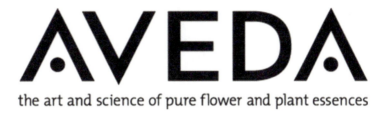

Joico

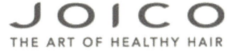

Avlon
KeraCare

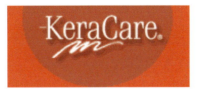

Mizani

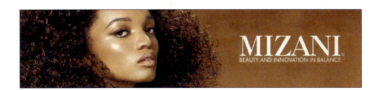

Paul
Mitchell

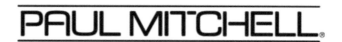

KMS

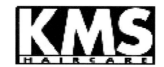

Any of these lines will produces great
results when used correctly.

Remember to stay away from high
concentrations of alcohol found in some
holding sprays.

Avoid the use of hair products with heavy petroleum contents on your hair extensions.

Regular cleansing and careful handling of the hair is the best way to keep your hair weave looking great longer.

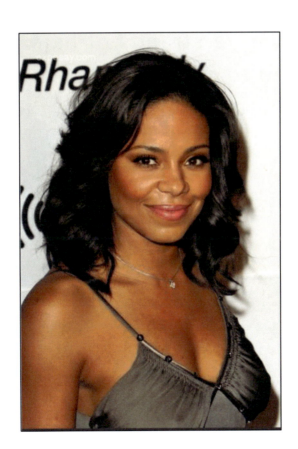

Vocabulary terms

Bonding: to attach wefted hair to the natural hair with a latex or surgical type adhesive.

Braid: to weave strands of hair together. This is used to form a base or track to sew on a commercial weft. This is the cornrow technique.

Cornrow: term used to describe an on the scalp braid. These braids can be used to form a track for the cornrow weaving method.

Hair Textures: European: Processed in straight, wavy or curly. Fine and smooth.

Ethnic Textures: Processed in straight, wavy or curly. More coarse than European.

Kinky: tightly curled hair.

Relaxed Hair: hair that has been treated to remove all curls and waves.

Synthetic Hair: hair that is made by chemicals. Artificial Hair.

Tension: stress created by stretching, winding, weaving, or braiding the hair firmly.

Texture of Hair: type of hair such as coarse, medium, fine etc.

Thermal Process: temporarily straightening the hair with a heated iron.

Track: a cornrow that establishes the placement pattern of wefts or strand additions.

Weaving: the process of forming a base (or track) along the scalp to attach wefted hair. This process is not limited to the cornrow method. Several other popular methods are the Euro lock, Microlinking, and Bonding.

Weave Needles: needles used in the weave process to sew wefted hair to tracks. Needles are curved or straight and very dull.

Weft: Commercial hair sewn on a fine base and used in the process of hair weaving. Hair is referred to as wefted.

Frequently asked questions (FAQs)

Q. What's the difference between hair weave and hair extensions?

A. "Hair extensions" is a catch-all term that includes hair weaves. All hair weaves are hair extensions, but all hair extensions are not weaves.

Q. How much does a 'professional' (full-head) Hair Weave cost?

A. Hair weaving costs for a full head can range from $750.00 to $2,500.00 for a quality hair addition.

The cost may range from a few hundred dollars to thousands, and will require $20-60 per track every 6-8 weeks for upkeep!

Q. What if my weave is too tight, causing me to have headaches or difficulty sleeping?

A. Rinse the hair using warm water on the scalp to help loosen tension caused by the braids. If this does not help, the hair weave should be removed. Weaves that are too tight can cause tension on the follicles and break the hair.

Note: Excessively tight weaves can cause traction alopecia, which may result in permanent baldness.

Q. Why is my weave shedding?

A. It is normal to experience some shedding of your weave especially if the hair is silky straight. If you notice shedding, you might need to add bonding glue to the weft the NEXT TIME you get a weave with the same hair.

Please do not attempt to apply the bonding glue to the weft while you are wearing the weave.

Q. What is the easiest way to get bonding glue out of your hair?

A. While this book does not recommend using glue in your hair, the best way to remove bonding glue from your hair is to rub conditioner on the affected spots. If that does not loosen the glue put on a shower cap and sit under a hair dryer for five minutes.

Q. What is a Quick Weave?

A. A quick weave, as the name suggests, is a quicker way to achieve a similar effect as a full head sew-in weave. Instead of braiding the natural hair, it's flattened and made slick with gel then dried under a dryer. A wig cap is attached to the flat surface and tracks are applied with an adhesive. Once the glue has set the hair is styled as usual.

Let us hear from you...

If you have any questions regarding the content of this book, our website, the products that are mentioned, or any questions at all, please don't hesitate to contact us at the following address.

We would love to hear any feedback on your experience using The Ultimate Hair Weave Guide. Let us know if you found the book helpful or have some ideas about how we can improve the process in some way.

Please contact us at:

info@hair-weave-guide.com

Made in the USA
Columbia, SC
08 March 2025

54842008R00062